WOMEN'S CHANTS
FOR UNITY AND STRENGTH

SUSAN C. GARDSTROM

WITH CONTRIBUTIONS BY

SAMANTHA KASMER
DANIELLE REYNOLDS
KAITLIN SHELTON

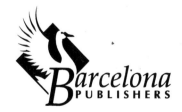
Barcelona PUBLISHERS

Women's Chants for Unity and Strength

Copyright © 2016

Print ISBN: 9781937440879

Distributed throughout the world by:
Barcelona Publishers
10231 Plano Road
Dallas TX 75238

www.barcelonapublishers.com
SAN 298-6299

Cover design: © 2016 Frank McShane

Dedication

To music therapy clients—
past, present, and future—
who amaze, motivate, and inspire.

Acknowledgements
☙ ❧

We thank the women at Nova Behavioral Health, Inc. in Dayton, Ohio for sharing their stories and wisdom.

Appreciation is also extended to Jessica Josefczyk, Tobias Rush, and James Hiller for their editorial assistance.

Susan Gardstrom
Danielle Reynolds
Kaitlin Shelton

Foreword

❧ ❧

Purpose

Most definitions of *chant* refer to rhythmic words or phrases that are repeatedly spoken or sung in unison by groups of people. Chants often function to support collective ritual. Some are celebratory and performed with great gusto, such as those we might hear at a sporting event; yet others are meant to be more contemplative in nature, such as those we might hear around a campfire.

The songs in *Women's Chants for Unity and Strength* are intended primarily for use with groups of adult women. Some of the chants may be well suited also to groups of older adolescent girls. In clinical settings, these chants have been used as a way to endow the singers with hope, courage, pride, and other individual and collective attributes and attitudes thought to lead to greater health and well-being. The songs have been sung to signal the start of a session, set the tone for meaningful time together, establish a therapeutic theme for exploration, and affirm self and others in closing ritual.

Although most were composed for groups of women who are recovering from addictions, the chants may have particular appeal for any person who has experienced the deleterious effects of abuse, marginalization, or disempowerment of any kind. In fact, the songs in this collection have been employed (both as is and with minor adaptations) in many non-clinical settings. Music therapy students in training, therapists at professional conferences, members of community and corporate drumming circles, support group attendees, church-goers, and participants in university wellness initiatives have learned and performed them.

No matter who the singers are, it is important for the facilitator to consider that singing, while a potentially unifying and liberating experience for girls and women, might be a threatening and even traumatizing experience, particularly for individuals who have experienced abuse (Austin, 1998). Thus, the facilitator ought to proceed with sensitivity and be prepared for a range of responses:

> Within a physically and emotionally safe environment, each woman can make an ongoing decision about her level of involvement: Some—too wounded to find their voices—sit back and let others completely guide the process while they look on and simply begin to feel again. Others select songs but do not sing. Still others dive in head first, singing fervently, playing, discussing the songs—even dancing—with little or no inhibition. There is ample room for all responses, and all are accepted (Gardstrom, Carlini, Josefczyk, and Love, 2013).

Contents

There are twenty songs in this collection. Each chant comes with a bit of background information and suggestions for performance. Next is a songsheet with a melody and chord symbols for optional harmonic accompaniment. Four songs include also a full piano score, designed for a moderately skilled player. Tempi and dynamics have not been notated; rather, these and other expressive elements should be determined on a case-by-case basis according to the intents, wishes, and capabilities of the singers.

Performance

True to the essence of chant, all of the songs in this collection are intended to be repeated several times (as befits the situation, naturally) and to be performed *a cappella* and in unison. Periodic modulations up a half step can add vigor and interest. If desired, simple vocal harmonies can be easily added to many of the songs. A few offer opportunities for solo singing.

A basic pulse or ostinato on a preferred drum is often a fitting grounding element. Piano or guitar accompaniment is not required but can provide harmonic support for timid singers, lend textural interest to the performance, and bring the energy in the room to an optimal level.

If the chant is unfamiliar to those in attendance, the facilitator may distribute the songsheets (for music readers), teach it by rote (using line-by-line imitation), or simply launch in, inviting the other singers to add their voices when and if they feel inclined to do so.

References

Austin, D. (1998). When the psyche sings: Transference and countertransference in improvised singing with individual adults. In K. Bruscia (Ed.). *Dynamics of music psychotherapy* (315-333). Gilsum, NH: Barcelona Publishers.

Gardstrom, S. Carlini, M., Josefczyk, J. & Love, A. (2013). Women and addictions: Music therapy clinical postures and interventions. *Music Therapy Perspectives, 31*(2), 95-104.

Contents

ॐ ॐ

Foreword v

1. Awesome Women 2

2. Be Yourself 4

3. Broken Wings 6

4. Come As You Are 8

5. Come To The Circle 10

6. Everything I Need 12

7. Here And Now 14

8. Let It Go 16

9. Many A Day 18

10. Many Voices 20

11. New Day 22

12. Now A Woman 24

13. One By One 26

14. Story of Your Heart 28

15. Stronger Than Ever Before 30

16. Take A Look 32

17. Take It Easy 34

18. We Have The Power 36

19. What A Beautiful Day 38

20. Woman Of Wisdom 40

Appendix

Piano score: Awesome Women 45

Piano score: Come As You Are 46

Piano score: Here And Now 47

Piano score: Woman Of Wisdom 48

WOMEN'S CHANTS
FOR UNITY
CHANTS
AND STRENGTH

1. Awesome Women
ॐ ॐ

Background: This song reflects that, on any given day, a group of singers will be characterized by tremendous diversity. This can make for a fascinating and rich group experience. It is truly a wonder and a joy that women with such distinctive physical attributes, personalities, and life stories can come together through music to form a common sisterhood.

Performance Notes: Although this chant can be performed without harmonic accompaniment, the thickly textured chords and "sassy" bass note movement in the piano accompaniment add solid support to the song's message. One or more participants may keep the pulse on a tambourine for added strength and timbral variety.

Lyrics:

Verse 1
Women, look 'round the circle, tell me, what do you see?
I see (seven) awesome women lookin' back at me.
Tall women, short women, big women, thin,
And ev'ry single one of us is awesome within!

Verse 2
Women, look 'round the circle, tell me, what do you see?
I see (seven) awesome women lookin' back at me.
Young women, old women, dark women, light,
And ev'ry single one of us is an awesome sight!

Awesome Women

Susan C. Gardstrom

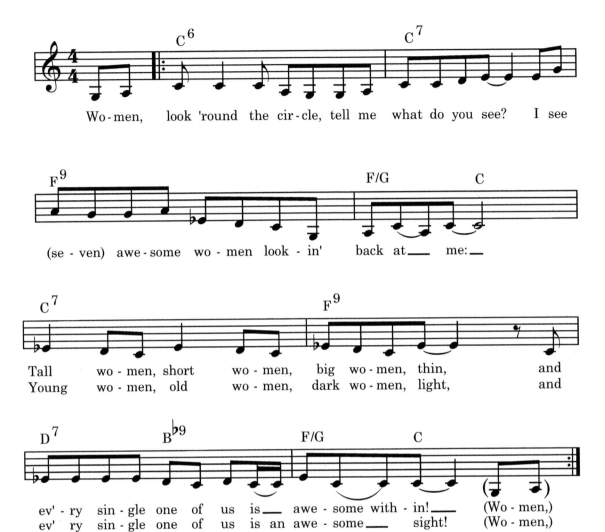

See page 45 of Appendix for piano score of this chant.

2. Be Yourself

↎ ❧

Background: This song was composed around one particular client's manner of complimenting others' appearance: "You be alright!" This short phrase embodies the notion that each of us is accepted and valued because of, and perhaps in spite of, our unique physical attributes. "Be Yourself" has been used both as a preface to and closure of exploration around themes of self-esteem and, more specifically, positive and negative body images.

Performance Notes: The leader carries most of this song; thus, it works well when, for whatever reason, participants need a minimal and highly directed role in the singing. Singers are encouraged (and often require input from others) to determine what makes them unique (e.g., smile, legs, voice); this is incorporated where the double stars (**) appear. The song ends with a vehement "alright!"

Lyrics:

Leader:	Be yourself.
Echo:	(Be yourself.)
Leader:	Don't be nobody else.
Leader:	Be yourself.
Echo:	(Be yourself.)
Leader:	Don't be nobody else.
Leader:	Be yourself.
Echo:	(Be yourself.)
Leader:	Don't be nobody else,
	'cuz nobody else got the (**) ya got,
	and the (**) ya got be alright!

Be Yourself

Susan C. Gardstrom

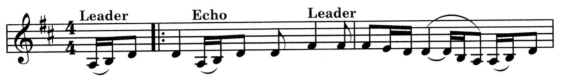

Be your - self. (Be your-self.) Don't be no-bo-dy else.____ Be your-

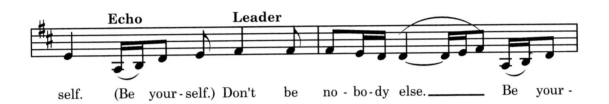

self. (Be your - self.) Don't be no - bo-dy else._____ Be your -

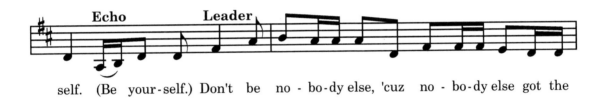

self. (Be your-self.) Don't be no - bo-dy else, 'cuz no - bo-dy else got the

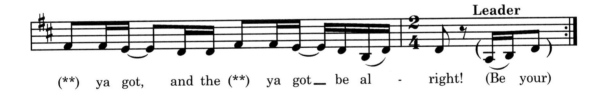

(**) ya got, and the (**) ya got__ be al - right! (Be your)

3. Broken Wings

જ ✎

Background: The catalyst for this song was an encounter with a wounded bird that was trying repeatedly to get off the ground. This was a powerful metaphor: Many women in recovery are like birds that, in spite of their broken wings, are determined to fly again.

Performance Notes: This song has been approached by singers both slowly and with great energy, perhaps signaling that different groups assign different meaning to the lyrics. Adopting a meditative stance, one singer noted that it "just felt right" to her to "pause for contemplation" by humming a verse before returning to the words a third time through. Adopting a quicker tempo naturally makes the elongated notes and phrases easier to sing.

Lyrics:

We are birds with broken wings;
We have endured some terrible things.
Yet watch us fly, and hear us sing,
This flock of beautiful birds with broken wings.

Broken Wings

Susan C. Gardstrom

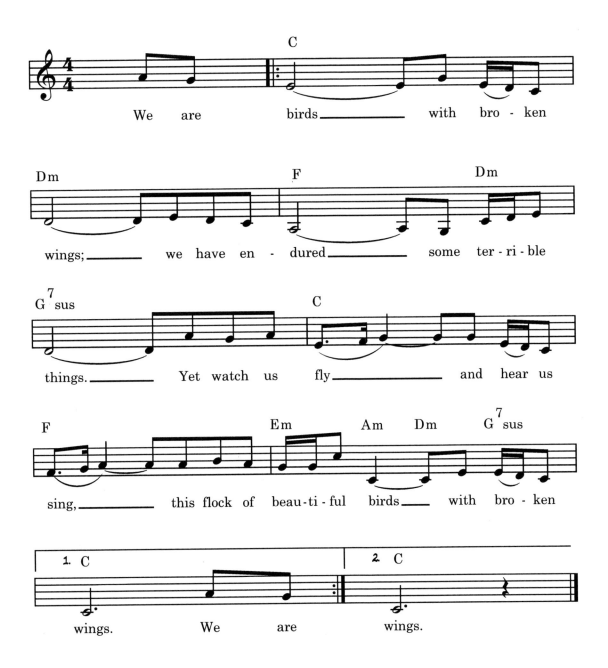

We are birds_____ with bro - ken wings;_____ we have en - dured_____ some ter - ri - ble things._____ Yet watch us fly_____ and hear us sing,_____ this flock of beau-ti - ful birds___ with bro - ken

1. wings. We are

2. wings.

4. Come As You Are

☙ ❧

Background: The main message of this chant is that the circle (group) can be a place where each person's "truth" is honored. In this regard, each member ought to be free to share whatever is in her heart, whether that is tied to positive circumstances (vict'ries) or difficult and undesirable life experiences (hardships).

Performance Notes: The melody is comprised of mostly step-wise motion, and both melody and lyrics are repetitive. These features should aid rote learning and recall. The chant flows nicely when the singers and accompanist(s) feel it in duple meter. With some rhythmic finagling, women's names can be substituted in the third, fourth, and fifth phrases after "we honor" (e.g., "For here we honor Larisa and Kim. And here…")

Lyrics:

Come as you are to the circle.
Come as you are and be heard.
For here we honor all vict'ries you sing.
And here we honor all hardships you bring.
And here we honor all manner of things,
So come as you are to the circle.

Come As You Are

Susan C. Gardstrom

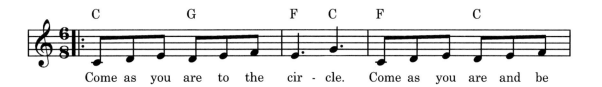

Come as you are to the cir - cle. Come as you are and be

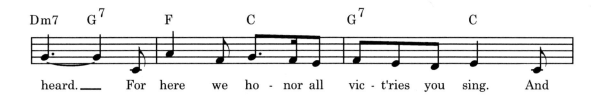

heard. ___ For here we ho - nor all vic - t'ries you sing. And

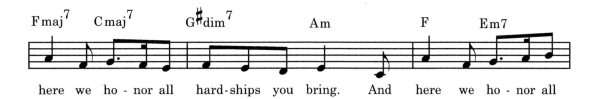

here we ho - nor all hard-ships you bring. And here we ho - nor all

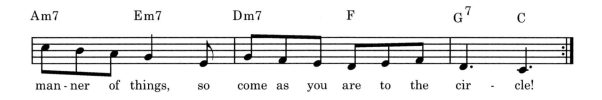

man - ner of things, so come as you are to the cir - cle!

See page 46 of Appendix for piano score of this chant.

5. Come To The Circle

‽ ‽

Background: When an individual joins an existing group—this occurs regularly in treatment programs with rolling admission, as well in support groups, certain social communities, and so forth—there is a period of adjustment, both for that particular individual and for the "veteran" members of the group. In short-term addictions treatment programs, this period is often abbreviated; that is, in order to benefit from the restorative aspects of group therapy, new attendees must shed defenses quickly and become invested and contributing members of the existing culture. "Come to the Circle" is an invitation, of sorts, to set fear aside, invest in heartfelt relationships with members of the group, contribute as one is able, and accept what assistance others might have to offer.

Performance Notes: It can be difficult at first to negotiate Dorian modality, particularly for untrained singers, but it does seem to get easier with repetition. This chant can be sung in unison or as a 4-part round. In either case, a single bass tone bar or one-chord (minor tonic) accompaniment can provide a tonal ground.

Lyrics:

1   Come to the circle, come without fear.
2   Join with the circle, let your heart be here.
3   Give to the circle whatever you can give,
4   And take from the circle what you need to live.

Come To The Circle

Susan C. Gardstrom

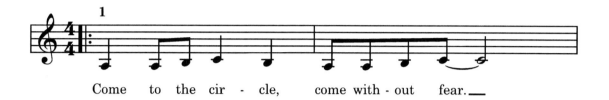

Come   to   the   cir - cle,   come with - out   fear. __

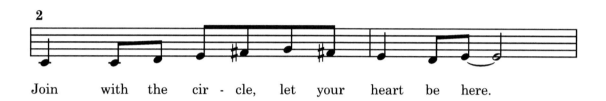

Join   with   the   cir - cle,   let   your   heart   be   here.

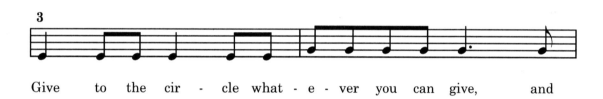

Give   to   the   cir - cle what - e - ver   you   can   give,   and

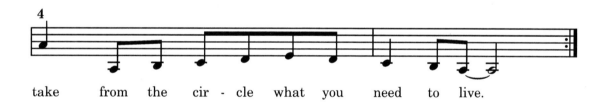

take   from   the   cir - cle   what   you   need   to   live.

6. Everything I Need

ॐ ॐ

Background: This chant aims to offer reassurance that each of us can access what we need to get through the tough times. For many women in treatment, this means *courage* to face personal "demons," *help* from family members, friends, recovering addicts, sponsors, and therapists, and *hope* that things can and will get better.

Performance Notes: This song seems to work equally well performed in unison with a simple ostinato or with piano or guitar accompaniment. The rests in the first ending allow time for breathing and ensure a solid start on the repetition—especially important when the first and last melodic phrases of a song are similar in contour. It is possible to adapt this chant by providing an opportunity for singers to insert their own words as follows: "I have _____, _____, and _____, and I'm learning _____."

Lyrics:

I have everything I need to make it through.
I have everything I need, including you.
I have courage, help, and hope,
And I'm learning ways to cope.
I have everything I need to make it through.

Everything I Need

Susan C. Gardstrom

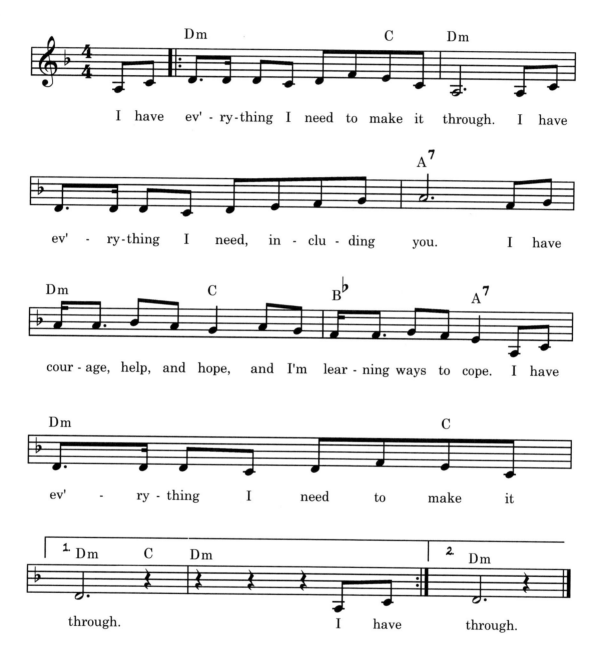

I have ev'-ry-thing I need to make it through. I have

ev'-ry-thing I need, in-clu-ding you. I have

cour-age, help, and hope, and I'm lear-ning ways to cope. I have

ev'-ry-thing I need to make it

through. I have through.

13

7. Here And Now

ಶ ೲ

Background: The difficulty of living in the "here and now" is a common thread in discussions among the women for whom this song was written. Wallowing in the past and, in particular, dwelling on previous failures, may lead to depression or a diminished sense of personal agency. Ruminating about the future may lead to feeling anxious and immobilized. This song's message targets anyone who desires to live more fully in the present moment, free from thoughts about certain circumstances and events in our past and future lives over which we have little or no control.

Performance Notes: Regardless of whether the song is accompanied with piano or with a single drum, observe the accent marks in order to lend both a sense of forward motion through time and an emphasis to the main message: "That's all we really need!"

Lyrics:

Here and now,
All we have is here and now,
All we have is here and now,
And that's all we really need.
Don't you know that yesterday is a memory,
And tomorrow will be what tomorrow will be. Oh!
Here and now,
All we have is here and now,
All we have is here and now,
And that's all we really need!

Here And Now

Susan C. Gardstrom

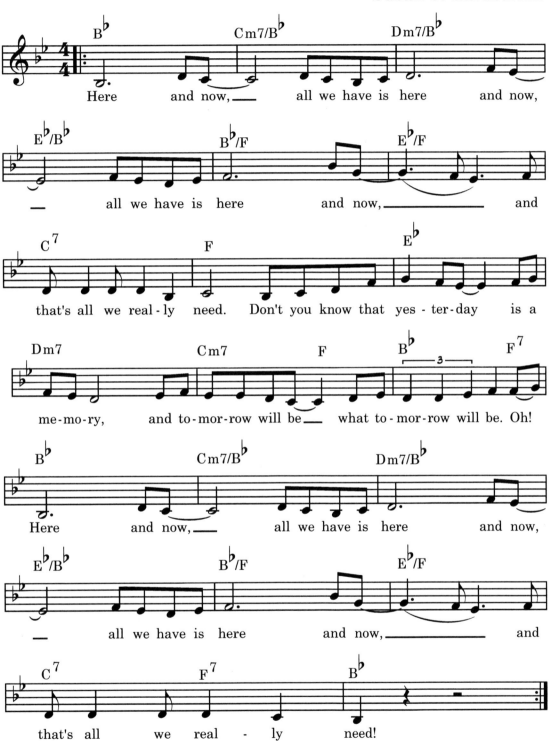

See page 47 of Appendix for piano score of this chant.

8. Let It Go

❧ ❧

Background: This song has a straightforward message: We all experience difficulty from time to time, and yet somehow we are able to consciously shed the extra "weight," make a turn, and move forward with new optimism.

Performance Notes: This can be performed *tutti* or in call and response fashion, with a solo singer beginning the song with "Let it go!" and the rest of the group echoing this line when it occurs (except for the final, elongated statement). Standing while singing and moving to the pulse seems to give extra emphasis to the song's message. Singers may add individualized gestures to the lyrics, "put your feet on the ground," "turn around," and "let it go!"

Alternatively, as with other chants in this collection, the song may be interspersed with percussion-based improvisation.

Lyrics:

Let it go! Let it go!
When the weight of the world is knockin' you down,
Take a breath, put your feet on the ground.
You gotta let it go! Let it go!
When the path of life isn't heading your way,
Make a turn to a better day.
You gotta let it go!

Let It Go

Kaitlin Shelton

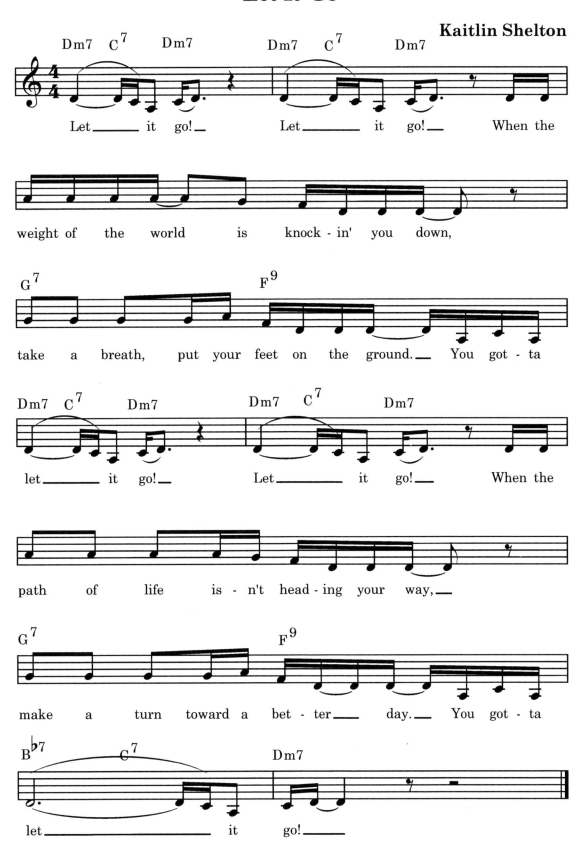

9. Many A Day

❧ ❦

Background: This is the story of the woman—any woman— who, in the darkest of times, was able to access something powerful enough to extricate herself from an untenable circumstance. Perhaps it was a co-dependent or abusive relationship. Gaining the strength and exercising the choice to walk away from an unhealthy relationship (particularly when real love still exists within it) is one of the most difficult yet necessary actions that many women take toward maintaining their own recovery and self-worth, not to mention their physical safety and that of their children.

Performance Notes: The extended measures (in 6/4) serve to underscore the importance of the words and give each singer a chance to breathe in between the phrases. Performing the song is thus a re-enactment, of sorts, of what a person would need to do—that is, take a deep breath before taking each of the challenging and often frightening steps that are described. A soloist could introduce the song by singing it once in a slow and highly *rubato* fashion, feeling her way through each phrase as she interprets the meaning. Once the group joins in stricter time, a percussive accompaniment with well-appropriated dynamic accents can assist the singers in navigating the unusual meter.

Lyrics:

Many a day I thought I wouldn't make it.
Many a day I thought I was through…
Then I raised my chin and I found my voice,
And I turned around and I made my choice,
And I walked away and I still rejoice
That I live to tell my story!

Many A Day

Susan C. Gardstrom

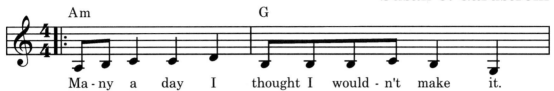

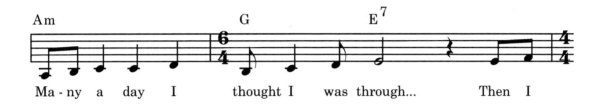

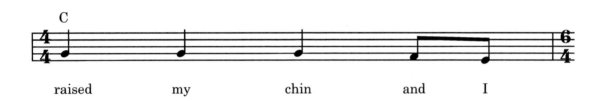

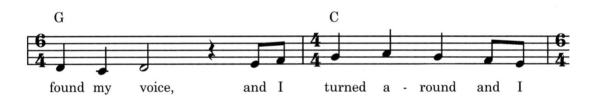

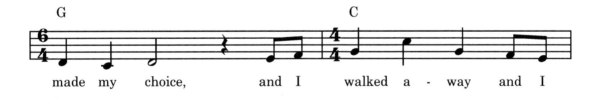

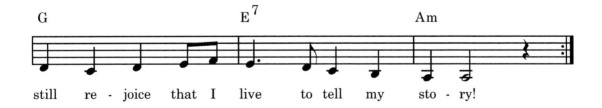

10. Many Voices

❧ ❧

Background: This particular chant flowed from a discussion about the many ways in which the women believed their personal freedom had been compromised, both through no fault of their own—many had been abused as children—and as a result of actions related to their disease—many had reluctantly become prostitutes, exotic dancers, and drug dealers to support their habits. Some residents spoke of a general reluctance to express themselves due to actual or feared retaliation, at which point the conversation turned to the notion that singing can be a form of collective expression, uncensored and unpunishable within the sanctity of the circle.

Performance Notes: With just a bit of coaching, individuals without past music training can render the two-chord accompaniment on a simple instrument such as an autoharp. The chant also can be "grounded" with single tones on a bass tone bar or open fifths on a bass xylophone. At the start of the second system, the first "Listen:" may be performed by one singer, with the second "Listen:" performed as an echo by all singers (or the other way around) to represent the individual and the collective.

Lyrics:

We are many voices, yet we are one.
Listen: (Listen:)
Women of the world sing a melody of unity and freedom.

Many Voices

Susan C. Gardstrom

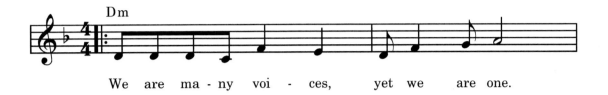

We are ma - ny voi - ces, yet we are one.

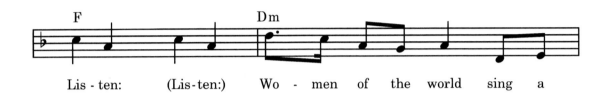

Lis - ten: (Lis - ten:) Wo - men of the world sing a

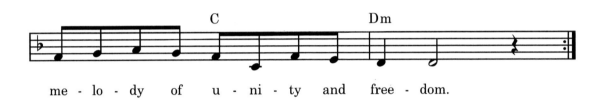

me - lo - dy of u - ni - ty and free - dom.

11. New Day

ॐ ॐ

Background: This is the chorus of a much longer original song from the 1990's. Because of its religious theme, the entire song is contraindicated for use with groups in a non-religious setting. The chorus, however, is a fitting way to reinforce the message that every day can be viewed as a new beginning with opportunities to make choices about how we will live through it. "We can take the wrong and make it right" evokes making amends, which is Step 4 of Alcoholics Anonymous (AA) and other 12-step programs.

Performance Notes: This song should be sung at a moderate tempo. The descending melismas at the ends of the first three phrases can be omitted if they pose difficulties for the singers. A steady and pronounced drumbeat may help the singers to access and convey their conviction.

Lyrics:

It's gonna be a new day.
We can live it in a new way.
We can take the wrong and make it right
And turn the darkness into light!

New Day

Susan C. Gardstrom

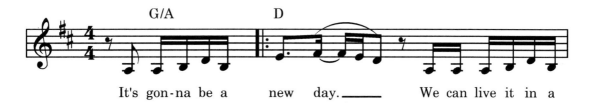

It's gon-na be a   new day._____   We can live it in a

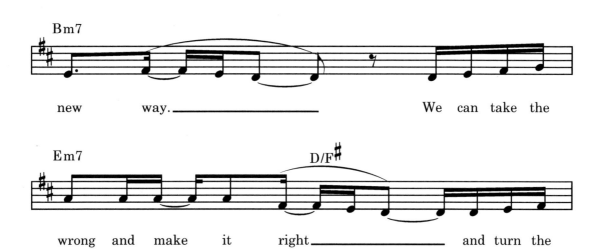

new   way._____   We can take the

wrong and make   it   right_____ and turn the

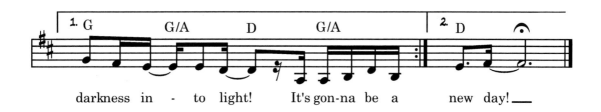

darkness in - to light!   It's gon-na be a   new day!___

12. Now A Woman

❧ ❦

Background: "She is ready for the world now!" was one woman's affirmation for another as the latter announced that she was "graduating" from the treatment program and moving into the next phase of her life in recovery. The first two lyrical phrases speak to the notion of recovery as a developmental process. The remaining lines describe some of the personal attributes that this particular woman hoped to take into her new world.

Performance Notes: The lyrics suggest starting softly and gradually building in volume to the climactic final phrase. A triumphant A-major chord (Picardy third) may be substituted for the A-minor in the final measure.

Lyrics:

Once a baby, then a girl,
Now a woman has unfurl'd.
She is strong and steady, caring and kind,
She respects her body and speaks her mind.
She is ready for the world now!

Now A Woman

Susan C. Gardstrom

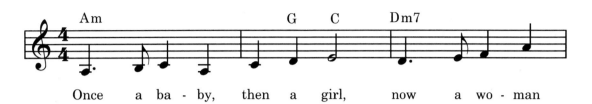

Once a ba - by, then a girl, now a wo - man

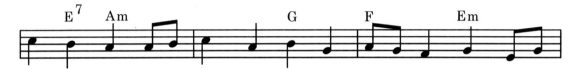

has un - furl'd. She is strong and stea - dy, car - ing and kind, she re -

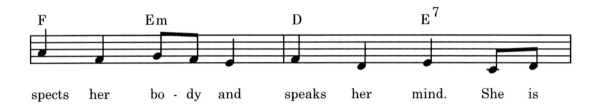

spects her bo - dy and speaks her mind. She is

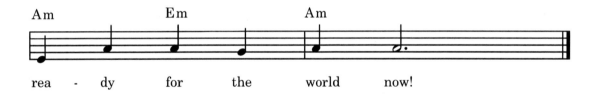

rea - dy for the world now!

13. One By One

☙ ❧

Background: This chant has no particular clinical genesis, but it has been used in a number of clinical settings. Its original function was to teach music therapy students a few basic strokes on the frame drum and model the use of song as a structure for rhythmic improvisation.

Performance Notes: Although this chant will work with any drums, it is meant to be performed on frame drums. Once the players practice a few basic strokes (i.e., dum, tak, cha, etc.), they agree upon a rhythmic ostinato to accompany the singing (e.g., dum-dum-tak-rest). The instrumental "afterthought" can be played on a treble melodic instrument, such as recorder or melodica. In the absence of such an instrument, the singers can perform this part on "la" or "doo." In between repetitions of the song, and for the duration of the piece (10 measures), all participants may improvise with drums and/or voices. When using frame drums and employing a thumb stroke, singers may use the alternative lyrics, presented below.

Lyrics:

One by one we make up the circle,
And one by one we make up the beat.
One by one we make up the music
That makes our life so sweet.

(Alternative)
One by one we make up the circle,
And thumb by thumb we make up the beat.
Drum by drum we make up the music
That makes our life so sweet.

One By One

Susan C. Gardstrom

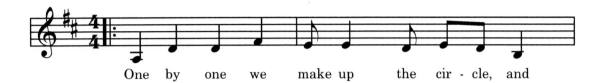

One   by   one   we   make up   the   cir - cle,   and

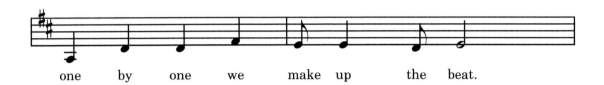

one   by   one   we   make up   the   beat.

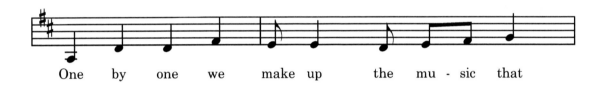

One   by   one   we   make up   the   mu - sic   that

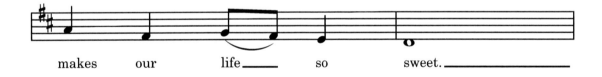

makes   our   life____   so   sweet._____

Instrumental

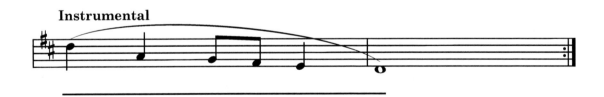

14. Story Of Your Heart

꼶 ꣿ

Background: This chant was written with the intention of leading the singers into a period of instrumental improvisation with a variety of drums (e.g., djembe, tubano, dumbek). The lyrics were generated with the aim of empowering and inspiring each woman to use her drum as a medium of expression as she lends her unique voice to the group experience.

Performance Notes: Prior to learning the chant, individuals should explore some basic drumming strokes (i.e., bass tone, open tone, etc.) and rhythmic figures. Then, the players might agree to either keep the basic beat or generate a simple rhythmic ostinato to accompany the singing. Singing the chant with accompaniment two or three times can then lead seamlessly into drumming improvisation for as much time as desired or indicated in between repetitions of the chant.

Lyrics:

Ev'ry one of us has a story,
And ev'ry story yearns to be told.
You can cry and rejoice with the drum as your voice.
You can play out the words
And let the story of your heart be heard.

Story Of Your Heart

Samantha Kasmer

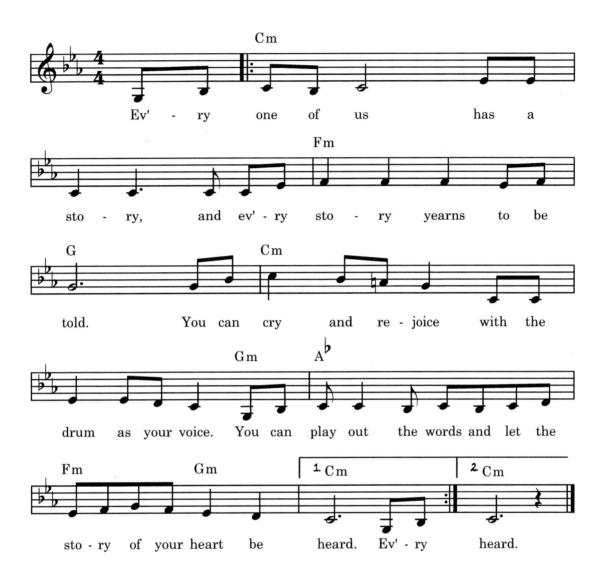

15. Stronger Than Ever Before

ఇ౿ ౿ఇ

Background: This chant evolved from a composition assignment for a music therapy course. The intent of the lyrics is to support the process of asserting one's uniqueness as a stepping stone to greater confidence and self-acceptance, as well as to call attention to the power of the collective female voice.

Performance Notes: As with another chant in this collection ("Come to the Circle"), it may take a bit of time for the singers to acclimate to the Dorian modality. Where "awesome" appears, the singers may substitute other words that characterize, for them, feminine power (e.g., wonderful, beautiful, positive). Ideally, because the lyrics reference a drum, each woman would be given access to a frame drum and taught a simple accompaniment pattern. It might be indicated to build in opportunities for drum improvisation in between Verses 1 and 2 or in between repetitions of the entire chant.

Lyrics:

Verse 1
I will sing to the beat of my very own drum.
I will hear the (awesome) power of a woman's song,
Steady and strong,
Stronger than ever before.
Yes! I am stronger than ever before!

Verse 2
We will sing to the beat of our very own drums.
We will hear the (awesome) power of a sisterhood's song,
Steady and strong,
Stronger than ever before.
Yes! We are stronger than ever before!

Stronger Than Ever Before

Danielle Reynolds

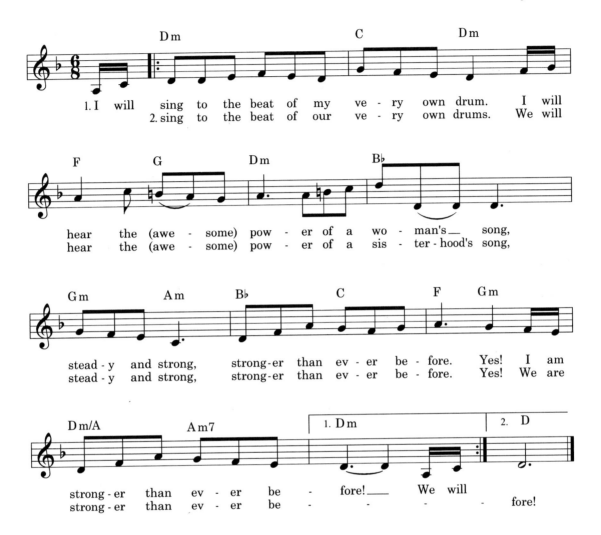

1. I will sing to the beat of my ve - ry own drum. I will
2. sing to the beat of our ve - ry own drums. We will

hear the (awe - some) pow - er of a wo - man's__ song,
hear the (awe - some) pow - er of a sis - ter - hood's song,

stead - y and strong, strong-er than ev - er be - fore. Yes! I am
stead - y and strong, strong-er than ev - er be - fore. Yes! We are

strong - er than ev - er be - fore!__ We will
strong - er than ev - er be - fore!

16. Take A Look

❦ ❧

Background: This song was composed in the 1980's for a group of adolescent girls and has been slightly adapted for adult women in recovery. The lyrics are intended to affirm each singer's beauty and worth and to give her permission to publicly claim self-pride.

Performance Notes: During the chant, singers may perform pre-determined body rhythms and gestures. The first measure of each two-measure phrase would begin with pat-pat-clap-clap (quarter notes). (Pat is performed with open hands on thighs.) Gestures for the second measures of each phrase are as follows:

Take a look – Place one open hand at eyebrows, scan from side to side as if looking around.

Picture book – Hold hands together in prayer position, then open to resemble opening a book.

I am proud – Pound one fisted hand on chest to signify strength and pride.

Right out loud – Cup hands on either side of mouth as if shouting.

If desired, improvised body percussion can be added to the song, with singers alternating between 8 bars of the chant (with or without the above gestures) and 8 bars of freestyle play, using a combination of sounds made with fingers, hands, feet, etc.

Lyrics:

Hey Baby, take a look:
There ain't no better in a picture book!
I love myself and I am proud,
And I'm gonna sing it right out loud! YEAH!

Take A Look

Susan C. Gardstrom

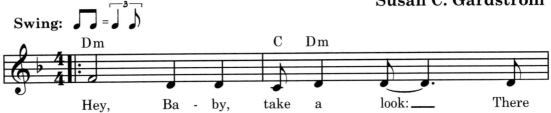

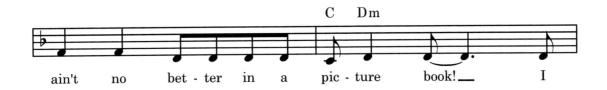

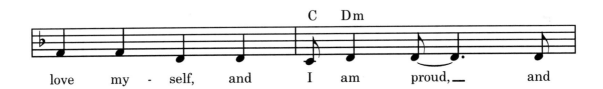

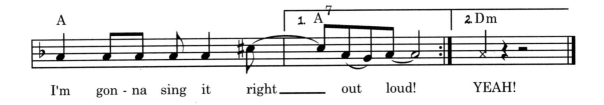

17. Take It Easy

ൟ ൟ

Background: Both in-the-moment anxiety and long-term stress appear to be common concerns among women. "Take It Easy" was created to prepare the participants for a session involving an extended music-assisted relaxation experience, which they had requested at the end of the previous session.

Performance Notes: One can sing this chant or, if preferred, focus on the breath and quietly listen while the facilitator sings. In the latter case, each two-measure phrase is used to regulate breathing, with an inhalation on the first measure and an exhalation on the second. Accompaniment should be legato. Tempo may need to slow slightly with each repetition in order to achieve the desired final respiration rate.

Lyrics:

Take it easy, take it slow.
Take a breath, now let it go.
Ease the body, clear the mind.
Leave your worries behind.

Take It Easy

Susan C. Gardstrom

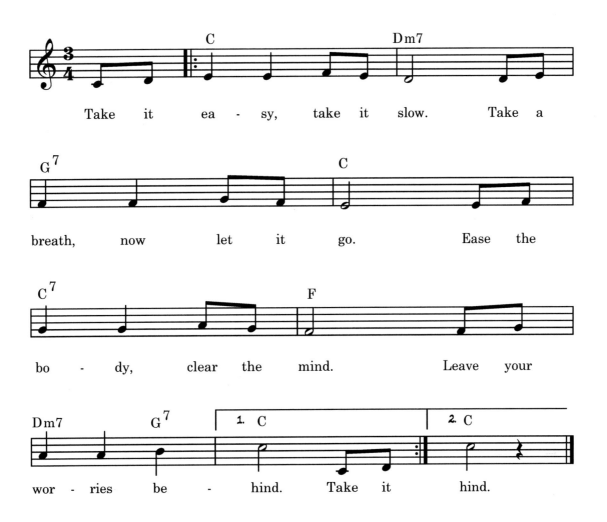

Take it ea - sy, take it slow. Take a

breath, now let it go. Ease the

bo - dy, clear the mind. Leave your

wor - ries be - hind. Take it hind.

18. We Have The Power

ॐ ॐ

Background: The message of this song is straightforward: Each of us has at least some power to create experiences of hope, joy, and so forth.

Performance Notes: The singers may contribute the subject of each verse. Favorites have included LOVE, PEACE, PRIDE, FAITH, STRENGTH, and FORGIVENESS. Some words, like the last in this list, are not easily positioned within the rhythmic structure of the melody. Nonetheless, all contributions should be honored.

Lyrics:

Verse 1
HOPE in this moment, HOPE in this day,
HOPE in this lifetime is the only way.
And you have the power,
And I have it too.
Yes, we have the power to make HOPE come true!

Verse 2
JOY in this moment, JOY in this day,
JOY in this lifetime is the only way.
And you have the power,
And I have it too.
Yes, we have the power to make JOY come true!

We Have The Power

Susan C. Gardstrom

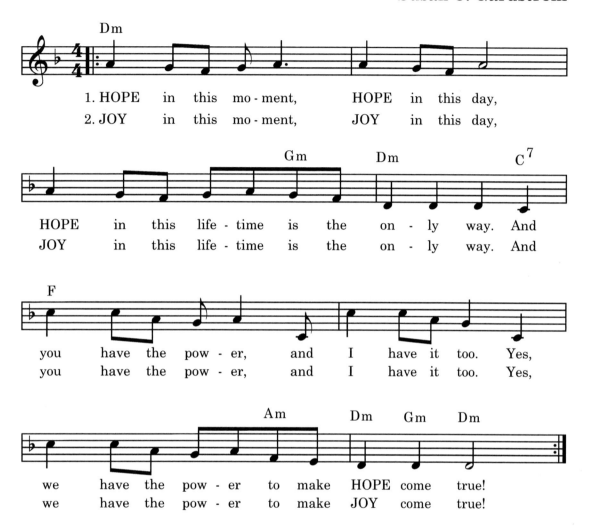

19. What A Beautiful Day

ک‍ ‍ک

Background: This song was composed to capture the simple joy that some women feel when they finally make it through the agony of detoxification and can see and think more clearly. Their bodies may ache in the aftermath of their substance use; nonetheless, they express delight and pride in knowing that they will be able to claim sobriety at the end of the day.

Performance Notes: This is a simple call and response song: One person or a small group sings a phrase and the rest of the singers echo. In groups for whom sobriety is not a focal point, CLEAN AND SOBER may be changed to WORKIN' TOGETHER, ROCKIN' AND ROLLIN' or any other relevant lyrics.

Lyrics:

What a beautiful day! (What a beautiful day!)
So happy to be. (So happy to be.)
What a beautiful day! (What a beautiful day!)
So happy to be. (So happy to be.)
Here we are, (Here we are,)
CLEAN AND SOBER. (CLEAN AND SOBER.)
We're singin': (We're singin':)
What a beautiful day! (What a beautiful day!)

What A Beautiful Day

Susan C. Gardstrom

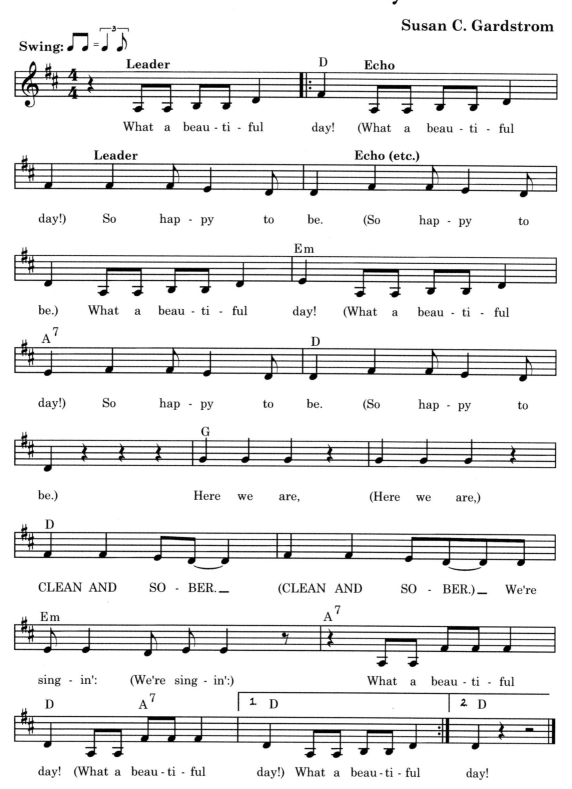

20. Woman Of Wisdom

ॐ ॐ

Background: To be sure, we do well to surround ourselves with people who lift us up—family members, friends, co-workers and other acquaintances who believe in our capacity to evolve into the women we are meant to be. And yet, the changes that we make are more likely to endure when we balance this support from others with recognition of and trust in our own inner resources. This chant is nothing more than a musical/lyrical reminder that each of us possesses valuable human resources, including innate and acquired womanly wisdom.

Performance Notes: The singers are invited to substitute "courage" with personal attributes and resources (e.g., "beauty"). If desired, the triplet motif can be repeated during the rendering to allow for multiple contributions: "A wo-man of beau-ty, am-bi-tion, con-vict-ion, and cour-age, a wo-man of wis-dom."

Lyrics:

If I could, then I would,
But then I can, and so I should
Believe in myself:
A woman of courage, a woman of wisdom.

Woman Of Wisdom

Susan C. Gardstrom

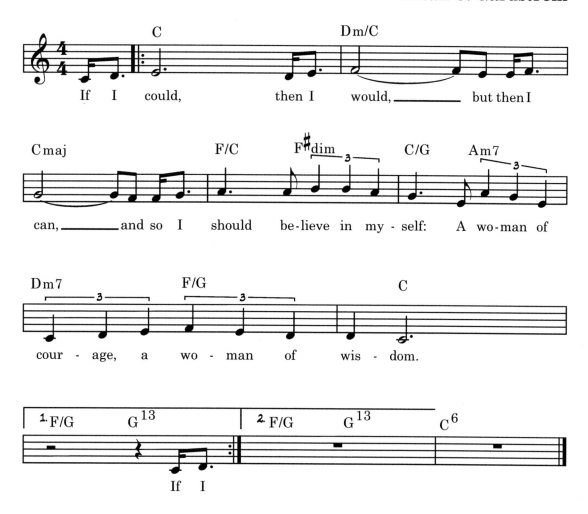

See page 48 of Appendix for piano score of this chant.

APPENDIX

Awesome Women

Susan C. Gardstrom

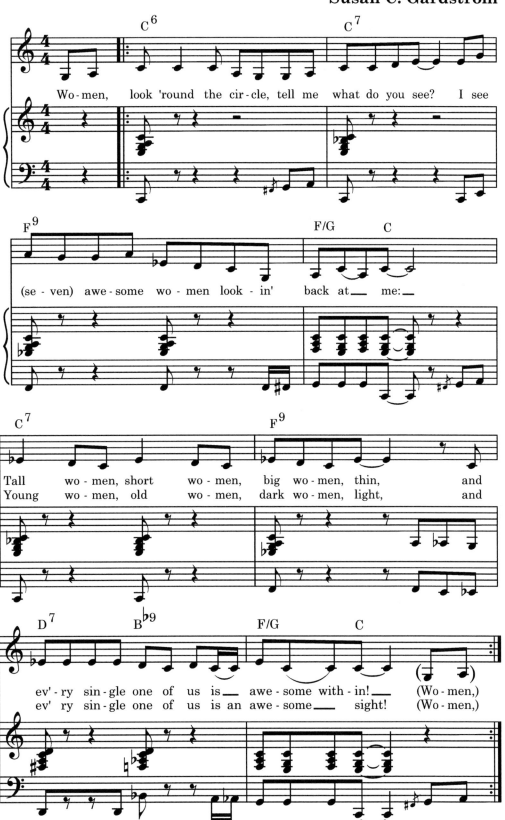

Come As You Are

Susan C. Gardstrom

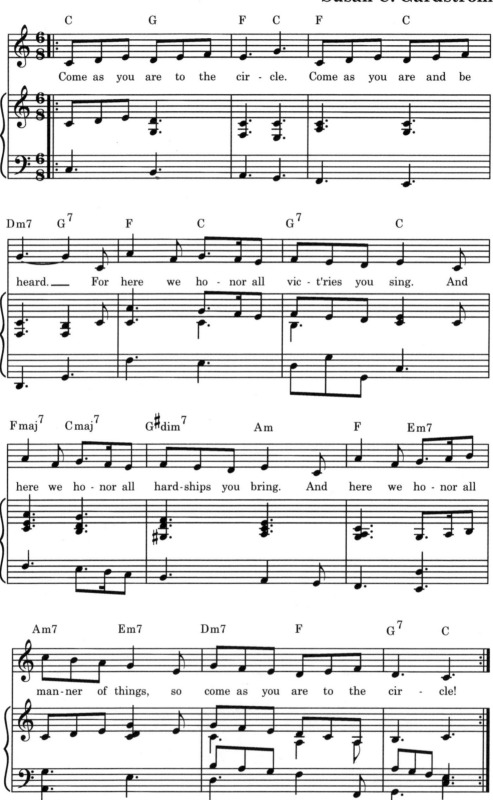

Here And Now

Susan C. Gardstrom

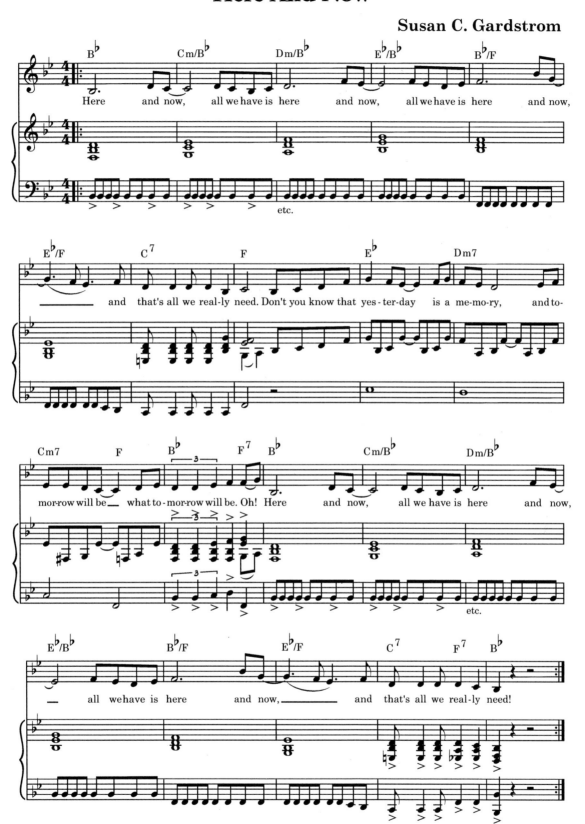

Woman Of Wisdom

Susan C. Gardstrom

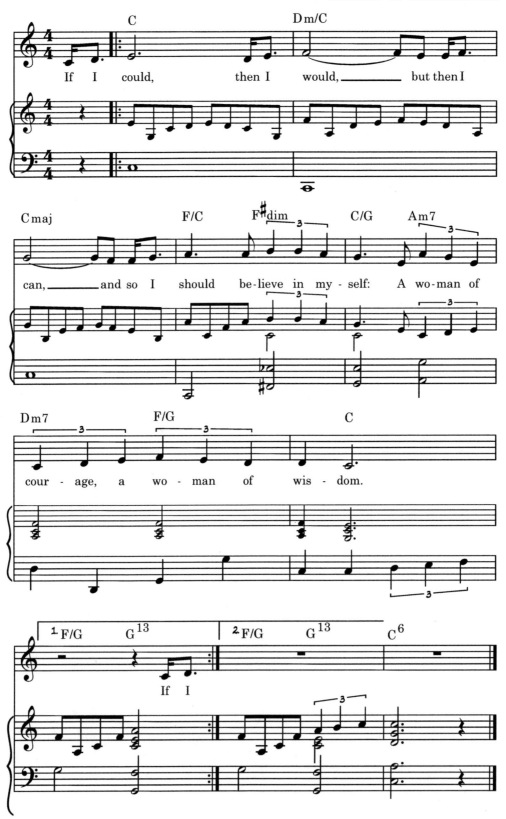

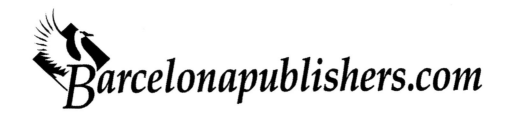

OTHER MUSICAL MATERIALS
FOR USE IN THERAPY

Composition and Improvisation Resources for Music Therapists (*Colin A. Lee, Aimee Berends, & Sara Pun*). This companion to *Song Resources for Music Therapists* is a collection of compositions and themes created by music therapists to offer innovative ideas for improvising and composing music in a therapy setting. (2015, 288 pages). Print. ISBN: 9781937440787 ($28).

Distant Bells (*Herbert Levin & Gail Levin*). Twelve folk songs from different countries, arranged for resonator bells with piano accompaniment, for elementary and/or special education children. (2004; 28pages) Print ISBN: 9781891278235 ($15).

Improvising in Styles: A Workbook for Music Therapists, Educators, and Musicians (*Colin Lee and Marc Houde*). A comprehensive workbook designed to give music therapists the tools needed to successfully improvise in their work. Each chapter focuses on a different style of music and begins with a discussion of its historical/musicological context and relevance to music therapy. Then follow exercises for solo and duet practice. Two CDs (or downloads) provide examples. (2010, Spiral bound paperback, 430 pages, 2 CDs). Print ISBN: 9781891278587 ($65).

Learning Through Music (*Herbert Levin and Gail Levin*). A collection of 42 musical activities designed for music teachers and therapists to use in their work with children of various ages, abilities, and needs at the primary level. With over 100 variations, involving singing, moving and playing instruments, these developmentally sequenced activities have been carefully crafted to help children develop: perceptual motor abilities, attentional skills, behavioral limits, speech and language skills, and relational concepts. (1998, 150 pages). Print ISBN: 9781891278006 ($28).

Learning Through Songs (*Gail Levin and Herbert Levin*). A collection of 16 easy to learn songs composed especially for music teachers and therapists to help children develop educational skills and concepts at the primary level. The songs have memorable melodies and lyrics that motivate children to develop cognitive skills in language, reading, classification, mathematics, science, and reasoning skills. At the same time, the beauty and structure of the songs help the children to explore their feelings and to develop interactional skills. (1997; 80 pages). Print ISBN: 9781891278013 ($16).

Let's Make Music (*Herbert Levin and Gail Levin*). Thirty-six original music activities and songs with classroom instruments for elementary and special education classes. These activities promote many basic skills, such as perceptual motor, language development, auditory memory and attention and limit-setting skills. Each child's response is simple and repetitive yet an integral part of the music, adding greatly to the child's success and positive self-image. And they're also great fun. (2005, 88 pages). Print ISBN: 978189127828-0 ($25).

Song Resources for Music Therapists (*Colin A. Lee & Sara Pun*). This companion to *Composition and Improvisation Resources for Music Therapists* is a collection of original and arranged songs by music therapists for music therapists. Intended to provide a diversity of repertoire for daily practice, the book includes: greeting songs, songs to encourage participation, songs to encourage energy, songs for self-expression, songs for reflection, goodbye songs, songs arranged for percussion instruments, and songs for music and movement. (2015, 230 pages). Print only, ISBN: 9781937440756 ($22).

Symphonics R Us (*Herbert Levin and Gail Levin*). Six original compositions of a classical nature for 10-30 classroom instruments with piano accompaniment, specially designed to give young children the opportunity to actively play an integral role in making symphonic sounding music. The music is thrilling and emotionally moving. (2006, 70 pages). Print ISBN: 9781891278419 ($16).